10 Habits of Happy People: Quick & Easy Steps to Be Happy Everyday (A Practical Guide)

SOFIE K

Table of Contents

Introduction

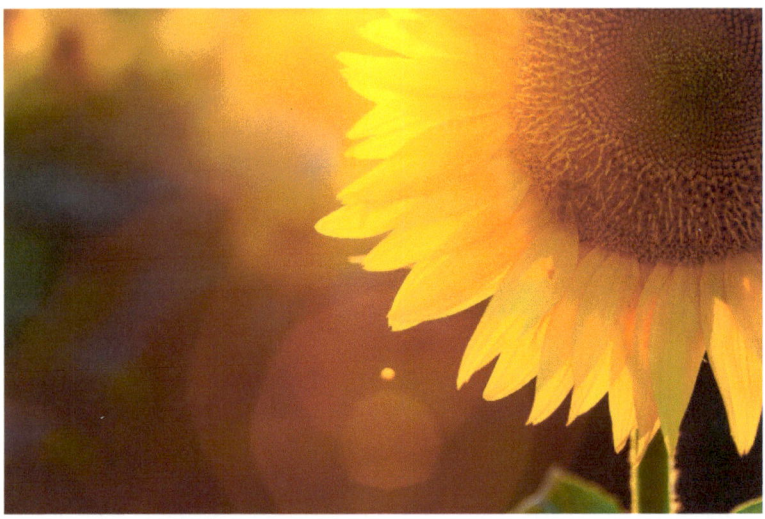

We all know what happiness is. It's that warm glow inside. It's uplifting, it's enjoyable and it is – according to many – one of the big things we're trying to achieve in life. And yet we don't spend all that much time being happy. A recent poll found that only 33% of Americans say they are very happy[1]. Considering that 39.6% of people will be diagnosed with cancer in their lifetimes[2] that is a shocking statistic.

---

[1] http://www.theharrispoll.com/health-and-life/Are_You_Happy__It_May_Depend_on_Age__Race_Ethnicity_and_Other_Factors.html

[2] http://seer.cancer.gov/statfacts/html/all.html

If so many of us think that being happy is a major life goal and yet so many of us are failing miserably at achieving it then something must be going horribly wrong. What could that be? Why is it that we do so well – and in fact ever better – on many other scores, like longevity, prosperity and affluence, but we do so poorly on happiness? And what can we do about it?

The good news: You can be happy. It is both possible and achievable. Yes, it will require some changes, both in lifestyle and in your mental perspective, but you probably already knew that. What's important is that these changes are within your reach.

We'll start off by exploring a common problem many of us have, where we believe we are pursuing happiness when in fact we're doing nothing of the kind. After that, we'll explore what activities and habits you need to cultivate to be happy. We'll dive into the different strategies, like mindfulness, exercise and socializing with people, which you can apply in your day to day life to significantly raise your happiness quotient.

By the end of the book you'll be forewarned and forearmed. And with that knowledge you'll be able to join that 1/3rd of the population that says they're very happy. What's more, in the process we might just be able to nudge that 1/3rd statistic a little higher, so that we end up not just being among the wealthiest nations but among the happiest to boot.

Chapter 1:   Why Be Happy?

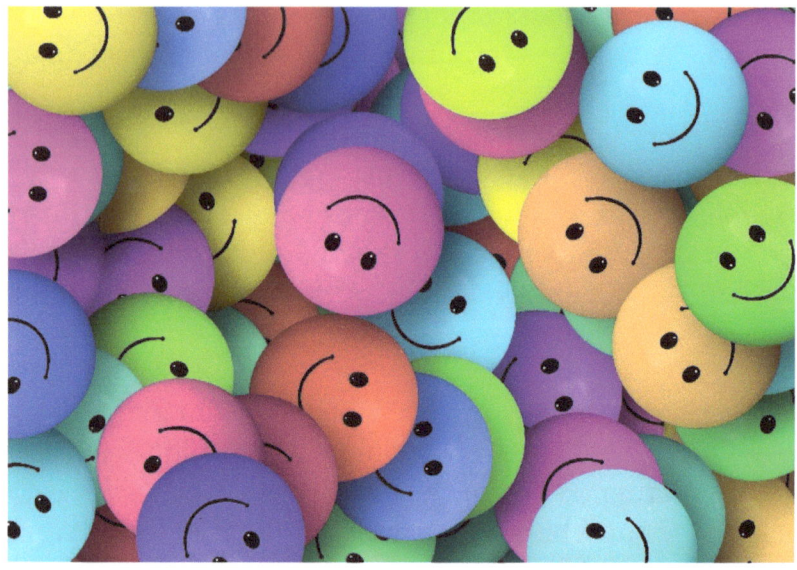

For most of us it isn't really a question. Still, there might be a few out there who've got a masochistic streak, who've lost sight of the reasons, or who simply like to know the facts. For them here are some of the benefits of happiness[3].

- **It's good for the heart.** Happy people have lower resting heart-rates and blood pressure. This isn't just short-term either, with people who were happier during one measurement still had better blood pressure three years later. In one test where people were rated in terms of their positive emotions at work, they

---

[3]   Taken from:
http://greatergood.berkeley.edu/article/item/six_ways_happiness_is_good_for_your
_health

discovered that every point a person scored higher on a five-point scale measuring wellbeing reduced their risk for heart disease by a whopping 22 percent. Yes, you read that right, for *every point* their risk went down by 22 percent.

- **It strengthens the immune system.** Happy people get sick less often. For example, in one study students were infected with the common cold and results conclusively showed that those who were happier got sick less often. Though the jury is still out as to why the body's immune system gets boosted by positive emotions that it happens is no longer in question. This might explain why when things are going badly you often get sick. Another interesting thought, feeling sick and feeling miserable might not be a one-way street, where the former leads to the latter. It might, in fact, be a two-way street, where the one reinforces the other!

- **Happy people experience less stress.** For most of us this should be reason enough to work a little harder at being happy. Being stressed isn't just a terrible feeling, it has numerous negative consequences[4]. And if happiness protects you from that, well, where do we sign up?

---

4   http://www.mayoclinic.org/healthy-lifestyle/stress-management/in-depth/stress-symptoms/art-20050987

- **Happy people experience less pain.** Being unhappy has been linked to feeling more pain. A study found that among women that had to live with chronic pain because of conditions like arthritis, those that were happier experienced less pain. Even more impressively, another study showed that people who rated themselves as happier actually saw their health improve over the following five weeks. That means that it wasn't just that their happiness buffered them from the pain like a painkiller might do, but it actually improved their health, like healthy food and exercise might do.

- **Happiness prevents disabilities.** The effects of being healthier as a result of being happier aren't just short term either. They've been shown to last. A study with 10,000 participants revealed that those who were happier were less likely to suffer from such disabilities as poor vision, strokes and chronic pain in the next 10 years, all of which are obviously debilitating. In other words, their happiness made it possible for them to get more out of life. And that means that if you invest time on being happy, you're likely to get it all back down the road!

- **Happiness lets us live longer.** In fact, not only will your life by healthier, you'll live longer too! In a noteworthy study, scientists analyzed the autobiographical essays nuns at the end of their lives had been asked to write when they joined a monastery in their 20s. Those who expressed more positive emotions in those essays lived somewhere between 7 to 10 years longer than their unhappier counterparts. That's right, their happiness in writing at 20 predicted how long they would live more than 50 years later! That's an amazingly powerful connection! In another study among the elderly, those who reported being happier were 35% less likely to die over the six-year period of the study. That's more effective than vitamin pills!

Fantastic, you must be thinking, I'm sold! Now if I could only be happier. But I can't. After all, happiness isn't a choice. It is what happens to you.

If that's your belief, then you're in for a surprise. This just isn't true. Yes, happiness can be influenced by factors outside of your control. Yes, it is true that 50% of your happiness is decided by your genetic disposition. But just because your genes and outside factors can influence your happiness doesn't mean in any way that happiness is something that is imposed from outside.

First of all, if 50% of your happiness is determined by your genes, that means 50% of your happiness isn't. It's a glass half full, glass half empty kind of thing. Secondly, happiness is a state of mind and though it might occasionally be hard to believe, states of mind can be altered. Admittedly, this is often a bit more involved than simply willing it to be so. Simply deciding you're going to be happy often isn't quite enough. Instead, you'll have to change what you do and how you do it. But it is possible.

The first step is making certain you understand the underlying psychology a little better. You see, we often believe we are pursuing happiness, when in truth were after something else. It is here that we turn next.

Chapter 2:   The Pursuit of Happiness

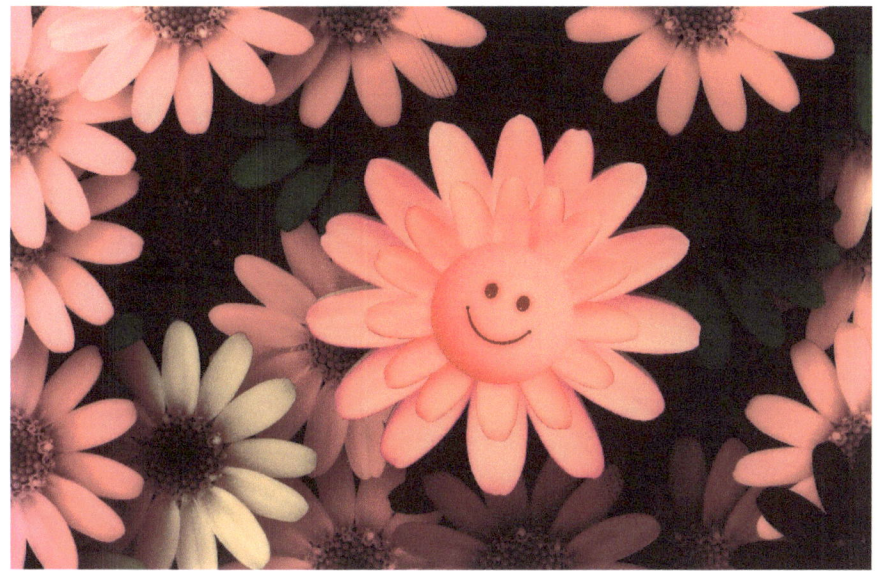

Though we'd all like to be happy, we're not very good at pursuing happiness. There are many reasons for this, but one of the biggest ones is that we're often confused about what makes us happy. As a result, our intentions don't translate very well into the right actions.

Research has shown us those things that are the most likely to make us happy:

- Spending time with friends and family
- Socializing with those we know and care for
- Relaxation and rest
- Travel and seeing new things
- Caring and giving (more so than receiving)

- Being intellectually and emotionally engaged
- Exercise and physical wellbeing

What doesn't seem to add much to happiness is acquiring stuff. Things like cars, computers, houses, couches, rings and expensive clothes just don't make much of a difference. Yes, you do experience a small burst of happiness when you first purchase these things. The problem, however, is that it rarely lasts. In their well-named research paper, 'If money doesn't make you happy, then you probably aren't spending it right' researchers Dunn, Gilbert and Wilson demonstrate that you get far more bang for your buck when you buy experiences rather than things[5].

If you look back on your life objectively, you might find this to be true as well. After all, how many things that you bought a few years ago do you still look at with a real feeling of enjoyment? And when you do get a little jolt because of some object, you'll often find this is because of what memories or what experiences you associate with the object rather than the object itself. In the meantime, when you talk with friends about happy experiences, you almost invariably enjoy it – in fact we tend to enjoy those memories ever more as they get further away.

---

5   http://www.sciencedirect.com/science/article/pii/S1057740811000209

So why do we buy things?

Are we broken? Is everybody that consumes an idiot? No, not at all. We just misattribute why we want things. Though we really believe we want them because they make us happy, we're actually pursuing status. Evolutionarily speaking, status is very valuable. People with higher status can influence other people to do things, can avoid being influenced and have a better choice of partners. All this translates into more and healthier children, which is the engine of evolution, with selection making that trait spread through the population. Thus, status seeking is something that we're evolutionarily inclined to pursue. (Want to know more? We suggest 'The Selfish Gene' by Richard Dawkins[6] which gives a detailed yet beautifully written account of basic evolutionary theory).

The thing is that unlike happiness, status is a zero-sum game. What that means is that whenever one person gains another person loses. This is because there is only so much mental real estate and when people are talking about one person, they can't talk about another. For that reason, you very quickly adjust to the status you have. That is also why you sometimes feel jealous when a friend shows off his or her newly bought wrist watch or hand bag. Any status they gain has to come from somewhere and that somewhere is sometimes you.

---

[6]   https://archive.org/stream/TheSelfishGene/RichardDawkins-TheSelfishGene_djvu.txt

This was actually tested. A group of researchers gave the equivalent of a year's salary to people in a remote village in Africa. They then explored what this did to both that family's status and the status of the other families in the village. As you would expect, the person who received the money experienced a status increase within their community. More importantly, the status of everybody else in the community went down. In other words, as one person gained, the rest lost. And so, because everybody is constantly struggling to gain status, we all end up running to just stay in place.

That's why the happiness boost from status-oriented purchases is only ever short lived. That also explains why when they do surveys about happiness, the people in western countries don't on average feel much happier than people in other countries. After all, in the struggle for status, you don't compare yourself to people that live far away. You compare yourself to your neighbors. And they're about as rich as you are.

Happiness, on the other hand, isn't zero sum. If you spend happy times with your family, then everybody that was there is likely to feel better. If you go traveling with your loved ones, all of you will (hopefully) enjoy it. If you're busy every day doing something that you love, then that will improve your days. And if you help people, then their gratitude will continue to make you feel good.

What's more, memories don't get worn like things do. That holiday you took to the Niagara Falls a few years ago is still just as it was then in your memories today. In fact, it's probably getting better over time as you forget the bad and enhance the good.

So should we stop buying stuff?

Not if you like the status that comes with it. And that is a choice you have to make for yourself. What you should do, however, is appreciate why you're actually buying something. Is it for status or for happiness? Status is a marathon that never stops. If you want to take part, you'll have to keep on running just to keep up with the people around you.

You can try to give up on the race but that is exceptionally hard. After all, evolution has instilled in us a drive to want status and when we choose to abandon that desire, we can feel like something is missing. In a way, status is a bit like sugar. Even though the enjoyment is short lived, it is very addictive. And like sugar you probably shouldn't give up on it entirely, as that's hard in today's world. People will think you're strange. Some will understand it, but for others the idea that status = happiness is a hard one to let go.

Instead, try focusing on understanding when you're pursuing the one and the other. When are you going after the happiness equivalent of a sugar high and when are you actually consuming something that's nutritious for your mental wellbeing?

Now, unfortunately, life's actions don't (yet) come with nutritional labels. But you don't actually need them, as with a bit of reflection you'll be able to figure out why you're buying or doing something. The question you need to ask is: *am I doing this to impress people?* If the answer is 'yes' then you're seeking status. Now, let me say this again, there is nothing wrong with that! Status can be very useful. It's a sort of unconscious currency of the social world.

What you want to avoid is becoming a status junky. You want to leave enough time, money and attention so that you have the time to be happy. And for that you've got to be honest with yourself. You've got to accept when you're pursuing happiness and when it is, in fact, your desire for status that you're satisfying. After all, you might be able to fool the people around you, but one thing you'll never be able to fool is your own emotions.

You cannot fake happiness inside your own head.

Chapter 3: The 10 Habits of Happiness

Great, so now we know what we shouldn't focus on. It's always good to know what you're not supposed to do. At the same time, it isn't enough. Based on what I've told you so far, dancing the chicken twice a day might lead you to be happy. After all, it's not seeking status and it kind of feels good. No, we need to know what to do as well! That's where we're heading next. It's time to explore 10 different practical and accessible ways to boost your happiness (as well as a bonus tip to avoid unhappiness).

Please be aware that some of these practices will be easier to perform than others. It's not necessary that you immediately engage in all of them. It's alright to start by picking the low hanging fruit first. Just as long as you start picking. Happiness shouldn't be a topic of abstract philosophy. It should be a part of your life. You deserve that much.

Acceptance & Perspective

"Whether your life is happy or not is your own choice. Many people think I can't live a normal life because I don't have arms or legs. I could choose to believe that and give up trying. I could stay at home and wait for others to take care of me. Instead, I choose to believe that I can do anything, and I always try to do things my own way. I choose to be happy." – Nick Vujicic

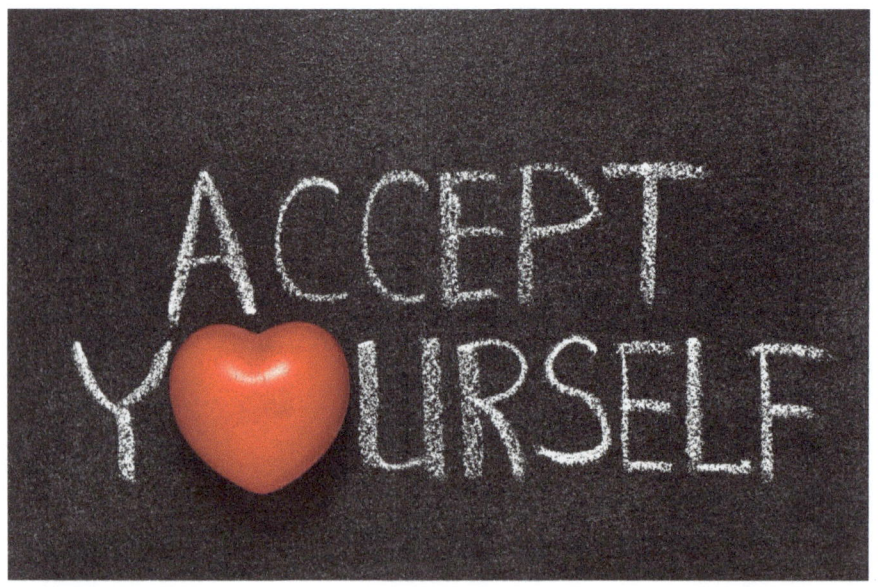

The first and possibly most important thing to realize is that happiness is a choice. Of course we're not suggesting it's as easy as choosing your dessert, but it is a choice. It is important that you accept that. If you do not, then you're taking on the role of a victim. Victims don't have any control. If, on the other hand, you accept that you can change your mental wellbeing, then you can take on the role of the protagonist in your own happiness story. You'll then have an impact on where your mental wellbeing goes and start changing how happy you feel.

I'm not suggesting that happiness isn't influenced by your situation. In the excellent book 'The Happiness Hypothesis' Jonathan Haidt demonstrates quite conclusively that this just isn't so[7]. At the same time, happiness is still an internal state and internal states are at least partly under your control. Again, that is not to say that you 'should just be happy'. It doesn't work like that. Instead, you need to change your behaviors, activities and practices and that in turn will influence your mental state.

Practical Considerations

One important aspect of changing your perspective for the better is removing people from your life who color your perspective black. We all know who they are – the complainers, the whiners, the hyper critical. We like to call them 'Social Vampires', as they suck the life and energy out of any party, conversation or situation. If we're serious about being happy we've got to let these people go.

---

[7] http://www.happinesshypothesis.com/

Yes, that can be hard. It might even feel like you're betraying them. At the same time, if a friend constantly cheats us by not paying for their meals and not paying their round of drinks, as well as borrowing money without paying it back, eventually you'd let them go as well, right? So why are you allowing them to shortchange you on your happiness? Don't let the social vampires suck the happiness right out of you. Take a step back and find people of a more positive persuasion to hang out with. This change alone will dramatically improve your outlook.

What if you're a social vampire? Then you've got to learn to bite your tongue. Happy people are a fantastic source of mental wellbeing, as they can offer you more positive perspectives and make you feel better about yourself and your life. This can often be exactly what an unhappy person needs to pull themselves out of a bad place. The thing is, happy people often naturally avoid the overtly pessimistic, as they don't want to be dragged down. So, when you feel the need to say something dark or criticize, don't! Keep it to yourself and avoid the negative feedback loop of driving those people who can offer you a better perspective from your life.

Giving & Serving

"It's enough to indulge and be selfish but true happiness is really when you start giving back." –Adrian Grenier

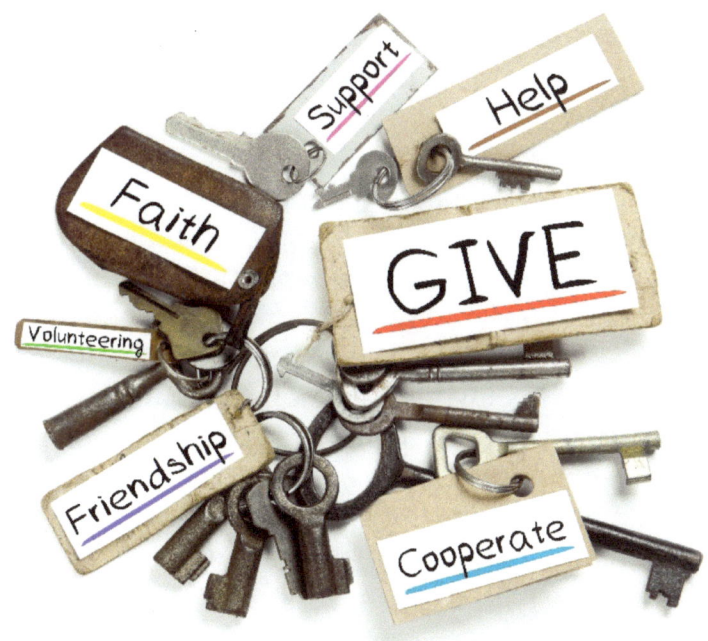

There is a small positive relationship between having more money and happiness. This relationship isn't a straight line, however (something that's known as a linear relationship). Instead it is log-linear, which means it's a curved line, where in the beginning the relationship is strong. After all, you'll be a lot happier if you're meeting your basic necessities like having enough food and being sufficiently warm. But then, as all you can buy is luxuries and slightly better version of what you already have, the relationship weakens steadily. And finally you need ridiculous amounts of extra money just to get a tiny increase in happiness. This happens much sooner than you may think.

A much more effective road to happiness than getting or receiving is giving and serving. Counterintuitive as it may seem, there have been numerous papers and studies confirming that in order to be happy, we should give to others. For example, those who volunteer experience much greater mental wellbeing (and live longer) than those who don't. This effect is greater than that of exercise and smoking! Similarly, when people were given a sum of money, if they then give that money away or spend it on others, they experience greater mental well-being than if they spend it on themselves.

The reason? In part it's obviously related to feeling good about ourselves. We like to think of ourselves as good people and it helps when our actions coincide with our beliefs. It also gives us meaning and makes us feel wanted. Possibly and most importantly, however, through giving to others we connect with them and as social creatures connecting with others makes us happy.

Practical Considerations

It isn't rocket science. All you need to do is give a little of your time or your money to others. You don't even need to immediately go overboard. A great initial strategy is simply to try to do at least a random act of kindness each day. This can be helping somebody on the street, paying for somebody's coffee, or offering to help somebody within your circle of friends and family before they ask for it.

Alternatively, do something more structured. There are always places that need volunteers. The act of scheduling in a period of giving can mean that you won't forget. This way you can turn the act into a habit and once that's the case, it's much less likely that it will slip from your life.

Some people find it very hard to deal with stranger's gratitude. In that case maybe try getting them to pay it forward? For anybody unfamiliar with this idea, it's quite simple. It's where you tell the person to help somebody else to pay you back and then asking them to pay it forward as well. The idea being that in this way helping is perpetuated, with each act of kindness promoting another and yet another. If everybody would just do that, how much better society would be! What's more, from a slightly more selfish perspective, if everybody continues to give forward, what goes around will come around and you'll get help when you need it most!

Relating & Connecting with People

"There is only one happiness in this life, to love and be loved." - George Sand

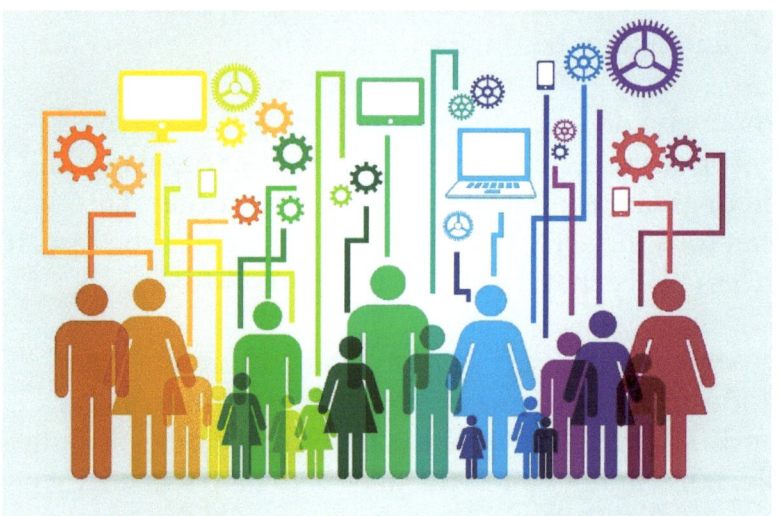

One of the best routes to happiness is to spend time with our good friends and family. There are no ifs and buts about it, spending time with those we like and love is win-win. It enhances your life and theirs. And this isn't just in the short term either. You'll have those memories to call upon in the future as well. And yet we often make the mistake of taking these people for granted. We let them slip by the wayside as we instead focus our attention on our work, our selves or our ambitions.

This is unfortunate, as the top one regret according to Forbes magazine is: *Working so much at the expense of family and friendships.* The thing is we all know it and yet we don't do anything about it. We wait until it's too late – when somebody's moved away to another state, or until they've moved on and we can never see them again.

What does the research say? The more interactions you have per day with people overall the more connected you feel to your community, which enhances wellbeing and protects us from negative events. But it is only the interactions with people that you care for, like family and friends, that increases your overall happiness. Of course, that doesn't mean you shouldn't interact with what are known as your 'weak ties'. For one thing, your weak ties are very useful for many other things, like finding opportunities. For another, you never know who is going to become a strong connection in the years to come! Just don't neglect the people you truly care about while you're doing it.

Practical Considerations

The easiest way to enjoy this type of happiness is to make certain that you reach out. This can be as easy as just calling somebody that matters to you every so often and having a ten-minute conversation. Maybe you've got a daily commute in the morning that you could fill with a call? Or maybe you like to relax with a glass of wine at the end of the day. Instead of watching TV maybe reach out to somebody?

The first step is obviously figuring out who'd you like to reach out. Make a list. A good place to start is with your Facebook friend list. Write down everybody that you've got, you once had, or you would like a good connection with and then simply start reaching out!

You can even use this book as an excuse. Tell them that you're trying to be happier and that connecting with people you care for is a surefire way to do so. For that reason, you're reaching out to them. Then ask them how they're doing and take it from there! Before you know it, you'll be reconnecting to people you haven't spoken to in years, planning to meet up with new friends on weekends and feeling that warm sensation of being appreciated and connected to those you love.

Another good way to connect is to regularly have dinner with your family and friends. Research has shown that happier families eat together. This allows people to strengthen bonds, share concerns and advice and have family time. It gives them a buffer for the bad times and makes certain that problems are tackled before they grow unmanageable. Note that watching TV together as you eat is not the same thing! The flat screen is only ever one way and therefore can never be a member of your family.

Exercise & Health

"My grandmother started walking five miles a day when she was sixty. She's ninety-seven now, and we don't know where the heck she is." – Ellen DeGeneres

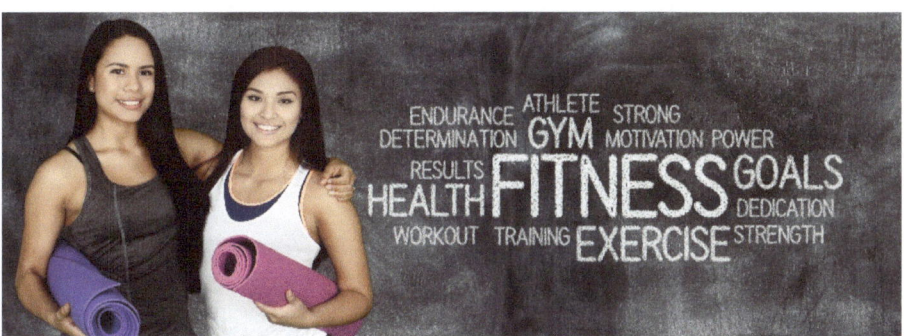

The benefits of exercise cannot be underestimated. You've probably heard all about how it boosts your physical wellbeing, but it doesn't end there. It boosts your mental wellbeing as well. It has been shown to fight depression, stress and anxiety. What's more, a good workout session floods your body with endorphins which pretty much amounts to a natural high. It also has numerous beneficial knock on effects. For example, you'll sleep better, be physically healthier and be mental sharper, all of which in turn leave you happier.

But you probably knew all that already. After all, they just won't shut up about it either in the TV or in the magazines. And yet, despite all the health benefits, there's a good chance that like most people, you're not exercising enough. After all, how do you square the time to get there, do your workout and get back to work with your busy schedule?

It's a good question. Here's another one: in a few years, how are you going to fit your visit to the doctor and the pharmacy as well as your sick days and your trouble getting around into your schedule? It isn't like you're going to be less busy. Rather, if the past is any guide, you'll probably be more so. Do you really think it is fair to your future self to saddle them with a dozen little niggling annoyances and problems along with what they've already got to do, especially when exercising makes you happy to boot? The question answers itself, doesn't it?

Practical Considerations

The big problem with exercise for most people is that they seem to think that exercise should amount to torture. Suddenly going from an entirely sedentary life to going to the gym every day is not the right way to start exercising. This won't flood your system with endorphins. Instead it will flood your body with pain as your muscles scream at you to stop hurting them. With this strategy, you'll end up resenting exercising in no time at all and that turns exercise from the enjoyable activity it could be into a chore. From there stopping is almost guaranteed!

Instead, take baby steps. Start small. Then ramp up. This way your body will adjust to your new routines and your muscles won't feel the need to murder you while you sleep. So if you weren't moving at all, then start with walking and riding a bicycle. If you were slightly more active than that, start running or swimming. Even just doing 10 minutes of sit-ups, pushups and jumping jacks is better than nothing at all. That goes double if next week you're willing to push that number up to 11 and the week after that to 12. In this way you won't just be exercising, you'll be progressing – and that's another good way to make yourself happier.

Mindfulness & Emotion

"Do not ruin today with mourning tomorrow." – Catherynne M. Valente

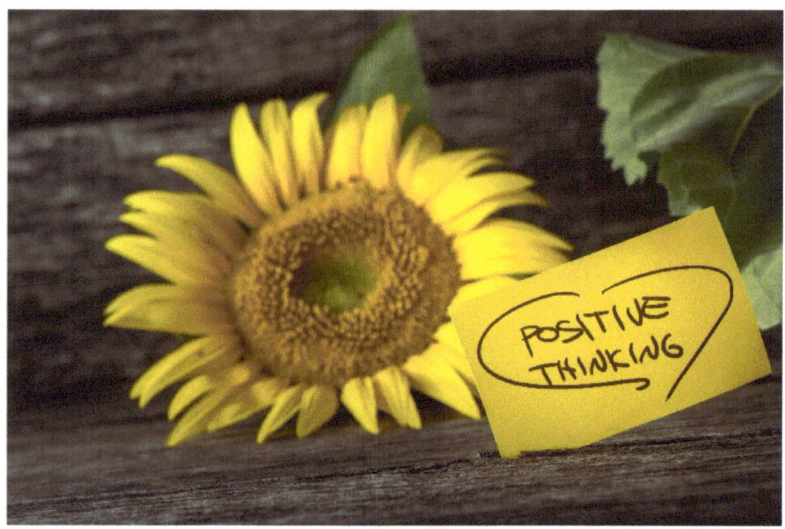

We are so busy with tomorrow that we often forget about today. Shouldn't we try to spend more time focusing on the actual moment? And that's not just for philosophical reasons, but also because spending more time in the present has been shown to have so many health benefits that it almost seems criminal not to!

Meditation – which is a fantastic way to train yourself to be more in the moment – has been shown to:

- Enhances happiness and wellbeing
- Reduce rumination and negative emotions
- Reduces depression

- Controls stress
- Enhance memory
- Increases mentally agility
- And so on[8]

For many, meditation sounds wishy washy, where eternally smiling people who don't wash or cut their hair talk about being a flower and understanding the meaning of a rock. We can understand why that might turn you off. Fortunately, it doesn't have to be that way. To practice mindfulness and meditation, you don't have to leave your living room and you don't have to pretend to be a piece of fruit.

All you need is a quiet space and some time. Then you just sit, focus on your breathing and try to keep your attention from drifting away. Even doing so for only five minutes in a row (which initially is surprisingly hard as we're not very good at sitting still) can be immensely helpful. From there you'll probably find yourself naturally increasing the time you're spending on it.

Practical Considerations

The best time to practice mindfulness is in the morning before the weight of the day starts bearing down on you. Sit down in a quiet place, close your eyes, clear your mind and focus on your breath entering and leaving your body. The goal is to exist in the present without judging it. You want to experience it without attaching either negativity or positivity to it. Instead you're just trying to be.

---

[8]   http://www.apa.org/monitor/2012/07-08/ce-corner.aspx

You'll find, in the beginning, that this is very hard. Either your attention keeps slipping and sliding or you'll constantly be judging your experiences. Don't worry about it. That's perfectly normal. Besides, one of the important aspects of mindfulness is not to get upset when something doesn't work out immediately. Instead, every time you drift away, gently come back to the moment and then try again.

An important thing to note: Mindfulness is not about progress. If that's what you're trying to do, you're doing things wrong. After all, progress is about the future, while mindfulness is about existing in the present. Mindfulness is not about wanting something you don't have. It is about being content with what you do have. In truth, there is no right or wrong way. The only thing you can really do wrong is to not do it at all.

The internet is full of resources that can help you practice mindfulness. A book we particularly liked was 'Wherever You Go, There You Are' by Jon Kabat-Zin. Alternatively, check out such resources as Psychology Today and the Berkley positive psychology movement.

Gratitude & Appreciation

"Happiness cannot be traveled to, owned, earned, worn or consumed. Happiness is the spiritual experience of living every minute with love, grace, and gratitude." – Denis Waitley

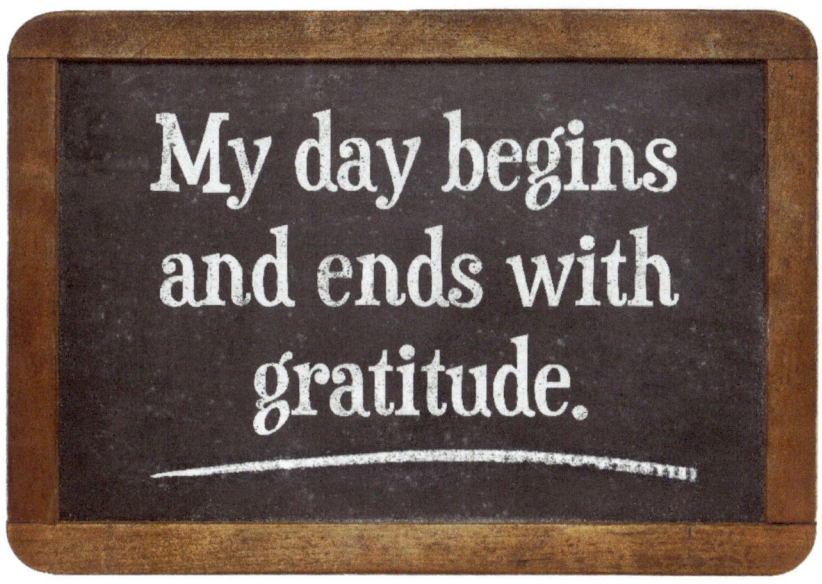

Want to be happy? Make sure to be grateful for and appreciate what you have. This is one of those examples where you've got to shift your perspective away from something you still want to something you're happy about, which can make that moment more pleasurable and can put you into a better mindset for the entire day.

How does it work? What you need is something like a notebook where you can write about something or someone (someone works better) who you are grateful for. Please do understand that this activity only works if you're actually grateful. Just going through the motions won't cut it. But if you can manage actual gratitude, the benefits of this practice are substantial. It allows us to realize how much of what we take for granted is in fact absolutely wonderful and that your life is better than you give it credit for.

You can write about anything that makes you grateful, really. The topics can be straightforward things like waking up this morning well rested, to something larger, like a family member, or to something more conceptual, like music, or sketching. One good exercise in case you're finding that you're not really experiencing gratitude is to imagine what your life would be like without that thing or person. Through the act of realizing how much worse your life would be you can often realize how lucky you actually are.

Practical Considerations

As said, gratitude needs to be real. Just going through the motions doesn't work. For that reason, it's important that you don't just write down a washing list of things that you're grateful for. Instead focus on something that matters and then spend at least a few sentences exploring it. Note that the act of writing is only there to catalyze your gratitude. The words on the page are a tool, not necessarily a goal. If you write a few sentence and after that find yourself reminiscing and thinking about how grateful you are, that's fine. It doesn't all have to find its way into the notebook – unless you want to be able to look back at it later, of course!

Equally important, gratitude journaling isn't something that you want to do every day. Paradoxically, the more often you do it during the week the less useful it becomes. This is because once you become used to doing something, it becomes less special and with gratitude journaling that means it becomes less effective. Once or twice per week is probably enough. It should be something you look forward to doing.

Finally, if you're grateful to somebody, think about expressing it. After all, as already said, giving is very good for happiness and that goes double for giving gratitude. People like to feel needed, wanted and appreciated. We all know that. And yet many of us don't say often enough how grateful we are to others for what they do. Often you'll find that just by expressing how grateful you are for somebody and what they do for you will strengthen your relationship and make both of you feel better about yourselves.

Do What You Are Good At

"Don't aim for success if you want it; just do what you love and believe in, and it will come naturally." – David Frost

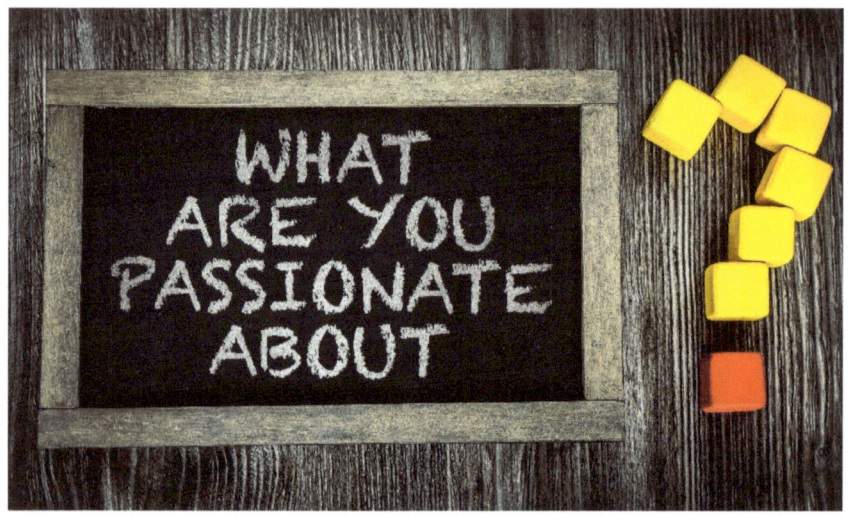

We like to do what we like to do. That sounds inane. Of course that's true! All the same, it is something we often seem to forget. With us allowing ourselves to get pulled into what we think we 'have' to do instead. That's unfortunate, as when we like what we do we take greater pride in what we manage to produce. What's more, we experience what in the research is known as 'flow'. This is where you lose track of time and your environment and get completely absorbed by the activity, allowing you continue for longer, do more and experience greater skill learning[9]. More importantly, research has demonstrated that this is a highly enjoyable state of mind to be in.

---

[9]   http://psychology.about.com/od/PositivePsychology/a/flow.htm

Now, that doesn't mean that you should throw in the towel and your job and embark on a life of artistry and poverty, but it might not be a bad idea to try and find ways to use your strengths as often as you can. Take some time to work out ways that you can more often use the skills that you're good at. This will make your working day more enjoyable. Shawn Anchor of 'The Happiness Advantage' had people figure out a new way to use one of their strengths every day for a week. He found that these volunteers ended up feeling significantly happier.

Practical Considerations

Sit down with a piece of paper and list ways that you can use your strengths more often. Be creative about it. If you're great at organizing, find new ways to organize your life and your work. If you're inquisitive, find ways to explore.

You can do this on your own or consult resources online that might give you ideas about how to change your daily situation. Another idea is to work together with a colleague, particularly if your talents lie in different directions. Maybe you can help each other make better use of what you're good at, so that you both end up enjoying your jobs more.

Then implement the practices you've come up with. You'll feel happier and, get to practice a skill that you're already quite good at – which will only lead to you getting even better and thereby enjoying it more. What's more, if you enjoy what you do and you're doing it well, you will get noticed and then you'll be a step further along your way to actively pursuing your goals and your dreams. And that, as we'll talk about next, is important.

Actively Work Towards Your Goals & Dreams

"The true cost of following your dreams isn't what you sacrifice when you chase them, it's what you lose when you don't." – Simon S. Tam

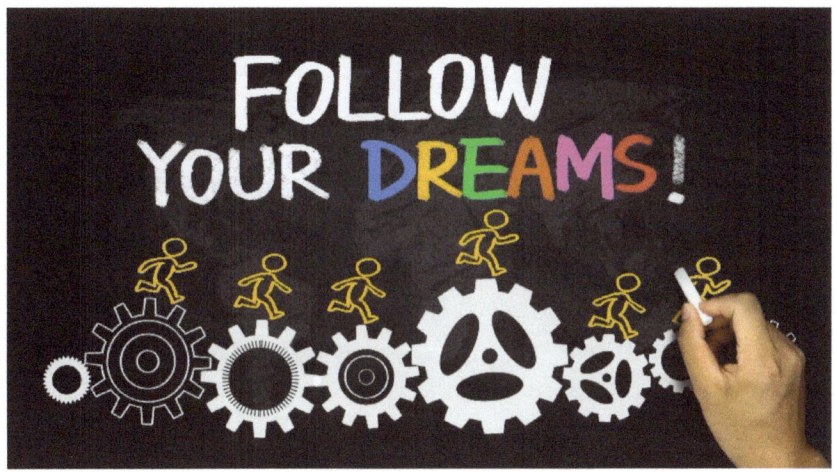

Are you actively working towards your goals and dreams? It matters. "People who could identify a goal they were pursuing were 19 percent more likely to feel satisfied with their lives and 26 percent more likely to feel positive about themselves," said David Neven of '100 Simple Secrets for the Best Half of Your Life'. Those sound like pretty good reasons to work towards your life goals. Another good reason is that you'll actually be achieving something and that you'll actually get where you want to go.

If we sit around waiting for it, life very rarely gives you what you want. It doesn't seem to work that way. If, however, you take it – well that's an entirely different story. So start today! If you want to be a singer, take part in competitions, join a choir and take lessons. If you want to be famous, make certain that you're out there, visibly doing something that can make yourself so. Neither activity will benefit from you sitting alone in front of the TV.

Another important aspect: make sure that you'll actually enjoy the journey towards your goal. We all imagine that when we've finally reached our goal we'll be elated, that nothing better will ever happen to us. That's unfortunately not actually true, for by the time you attain your goal you'll long since have adjusted to nearly having done so.

What do I mean with that? When you write a book you don't go suddenly from not having a single word to having completed a manuscript. Similarly, very few people go from being poor to being rich in one leap. You have to pass through all the in between stages as well – so less poor, well off, quite rich, and so on. And as you get closer and closer you'll get used to where you are and adjust your expectations accordingly. So when you write that last word, or make that final dollar, it isn't some giant leap, like you're imagining today, but rather just a final step on a long road. Yes, you'll be pleased, but elated is a strong word. Instead you'll get your enjoyment in pursuing your goals from one day to the next – you'll enjoy having finished another chapter, or having made a good deal.

With this in mind, make sure you set up goals that you'll enjoy working towards. Make sure that you can enjoy the journey itself. That way you'll get even more enjoyment from pursuing your goals.

Practical Considerations

The difference between goals and dreams is that dreams exist somewhere in the distance, hazily connected to your life only by your wants. Goals, on the other hands, have detailed plans to get you from here to there. The former lends itself well to wishful thinking. The latter, in the meantime, lends itself far better to actual implementation. So make sure you're pursuing goals, not dreams. Take the time to write out a plan, or draft a route. Consult biographies, business books and websites. Find out what other people have done, so that you can learn from their mistakes.

And then write it down. It doesn't have to be master plan. Heck, write it on the back of a napkin if you want to. It can be rough and you can certainly change it. The very act of writing it down, however, has the advantages of forcing you to think about what you need to do in a more structured manner and realize some of the unseen pitfalls that threaten your goals.

And you know what? Even just the act of starting to work on a plan and figure out what steps you have to take might help to make you happier. After all, you're now being active in the pursuit of your plan, rather than just passively waiting for things to happen. And yes, it might be a long road, but the simple act of progressing already has benefits, so that's not necessarily a bad thing.

Also, remember to be flexible. Nothing has to be written in stone. As the situation on the ground shifts or your understanding of how things work changes, your plan should change as well. Even your goals might shift. There's nothing wrong with that. Just be sure to look back to your plan often, and to modify and change what you've still got to do. As an added bonus, doing this will help you see what you've already done. Perhaps that's something you can be grateful for.

Be Part of Something Bigger & find Meaning

"When you become part of something, in some way you count. It could be a march; it could be a rally, even a brief one. You're part of something, and you suddenly realize you count. To count is very important." – Studs Terkel

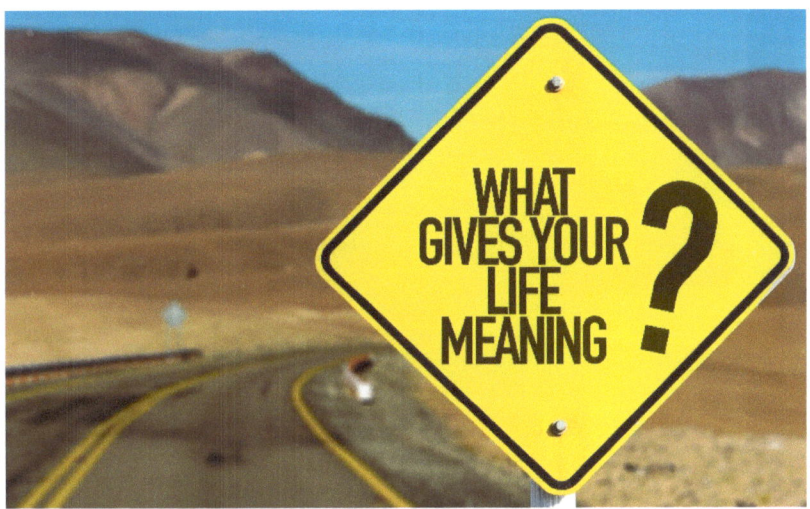

Being part of something bigger, like a faith, a charity, or a company, can lead to you feeling like you're more in control of your life and will protect you against such things as stress, anxiety and depression[10]. For this reason, people that have faith are on average happier than those without, both because of the meaning and because they get to be part of a community of like-minded people who are after the same thing.

---

[10] http://www.actionforhappiness.org/10-keys-to-happier-living/be-part-of-something-bigger/details

This is not the only way to find meaning, however. You can also find meaning in your job or your calling. If you feel you're doing what you were put here for, that often will also satisfy your desire for meaning and boost your happiness. This is in part why it's so good for us to devote time to what we're good at – it won't just satisfy us at that moment, but if we can become good enough, it can lead to us feeling our lives are more important than just waking up in the morning and going to be bed at night.

Meaning seems to be important, because as social creature we like to lose ourselves either in groups, or in concepts that are bigger than ourselves. Jonathan Haidt talks about getting consumed by something bigger than yourself as getting in touched with divinity – religious or otherwise – which is a step above the normal and the mundane and makes us feel better than we actually are.

Practical Considerations

Unfortunately, though having meaning is brilliant, getting there can be hard. You can't force meaning. However much you might want something to give you meaning, if it doesn't, it doesn't. That is a hard thing to change. You probably shouldn't try, as research seems to indicate that those who search too hard for their meaning have a higher risk of ending up anxious and depressed.

The search for meaning is better approached sideways, through one of the other activities we've mentioned so far. Many people find meaning in friends, family, meditation or pursuing their dreams, to name but a few. Simply try to be open to it.

However, you go about doing it, you have to let life show you the way. And when there is an opportunity to find meaning, you should be willing to embrace it. Don't sacrifice meaning to materialism. The research is pretty unforgiving about this. Though in the short term you might experience a happiness boost, in the end you'll be filled with regret for what you've lost. For those who pursue something immaterial, like purpose and identity, report more life-satisfaction than those who pursue material things instead.

Resilience

"When the going gets tough, the tough get going." – Idiom

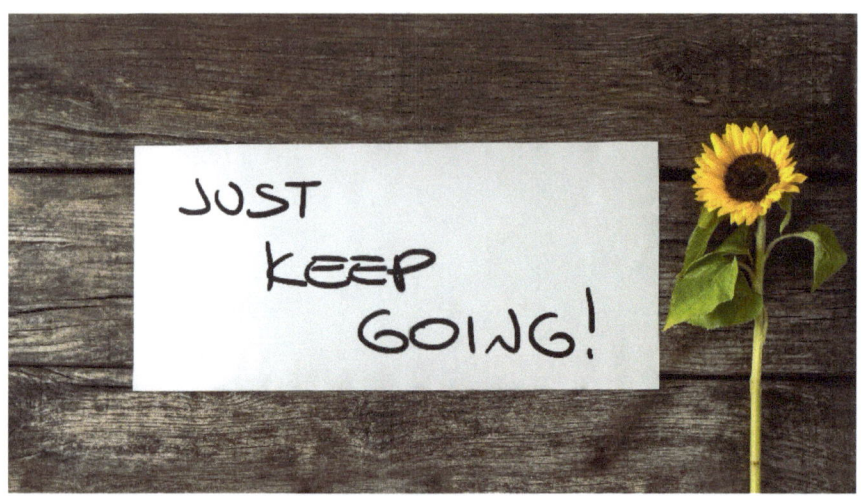

Resilience doesn't directly contribute to your happiness. Instead, when you have it, you reduce the fragility of your happiness; and that, is equally important. Sometimes life is hard. That's just how it is. What's important is that you have the wherewithal to deal with it when it does get tough. According to Peter Kramer, author of 'Against Depression' and 'Listening to Prozac' it isn't happiness, but emotional resilience that is the opposite of depression.

If you've got the ability to absorb emotional shocks, then you're in a better position to not ended up been swallowed by unhappiness when bad things happen. Instead you'll be able to bounce back and continue living your life positively. In these cases, the misfortune is nothing more than a bump in the road that is quickly forgotten.

If you don't have any emotional resilience, however, and your happiness is brittle, then even a minor upset might provoke a mental breakdown. At this point your belief that everything is going horrible might well become a self-fulfilling prophecy, as your actions and your choices create more and more problems. And then it becomes ever more difficult to lift yourself back out again.

So how do you become emotionally resilient? Do you need to practice another whole set of habits and strategies? Fortunately, no. A lot of the things we've already mentioned contribute to emotional resilience. Here we'll list some examples, to help you work on this important mental facet and keep your happiness on track:

- **Get enough sleep** – a tired brain is an irrational brain. If you don't get enough sleep you're more likely to ruminate and less able to regulate your emotions.

- **Eat right** – try to avoid nicotine, caffeine, alcohol, sugar, white flour, and processed food. Try to eat more protein, minerals, omage-3, whole grains, beans, potatoes, vegetables and vitamins of the B-complex, as well as C, D, and E.

- **Exercise** – As already mentioned, exercise is essential for a well-balanced mental state.

- **Maintain good relationships** – Not only do friends, family and loved ones make you happier but they also offer a buffer against the world's woes. You can talk to them about your problems and they can offer you advice, resources or support to help you overcome them.

- **Purpose** – if you're working towards something or part of something that you think is important, this can give you the will to continue when the going gets tough.

- **Gratitude** – if you know what you're happy about, this will protect you from sadness and will give you reason to work harder to keep on track and protect what you already have. In this way gratitude doesn't just make you happier, but makes you more resilient as well.

Practical Considerations

The Social psychologist Roy Baumeister famously said, "Bad is stronger than good". With that he didn't mean that it was in any way better, but rather that in our minds it weighs more heavily. And with good reason. For example, if I offered you a coin toss to either double all the money you have or lose all the money you have, you'd probably not take it. After all, though doubling your money is nice, perhaps even very nice, the consequences of losing it all would be devastating.

Similarly, though becoming happy is wonderful, if you become unhappy or depressed that will be far more debilitating. For that reason, it is important that you make sure that you don't just work at being happier, but that you also work at being more resilience so that you can weather the storms when they come and you can maintain a positive perspective.

Conclusion

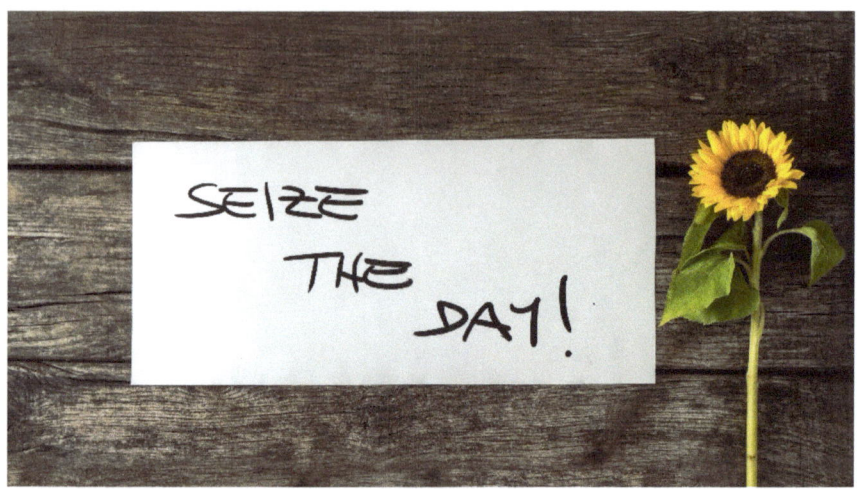

Happiness isn't a destination. Nor is it a decision. Instead, much like life, it is a work in progress. It's a matter of laying the right foundation, then building continuously on top of that. This book has been directed at giving you exactly that. If you refine your focus away from status and towards happiness, as well as practicing the 10 + 1 habits that we've outlined here, your mental wellbeing will improve. The research backs that up.

What's more, the habits of happiness aren't even that hard, nor do they require, drugs, medicine or any weird voodoo-like rituals. In large parts, it's a matter of doing those things that we all already know are healthy for us, but have somehow fallen by the wayside over the last century or so.

To be happy we first of all have to make sure we're focusing on the right thing. Then we've got to accept that happiness is a synergy between your mind, your feelings and your body. It's a combination of practices and beliefs. It isn't hocus-pocus. Instead it is a matter of having the correct focus. In truth, what seems to have happened is that as we've advanced, we've lost sight of the path to happiness.

In a nutshell, we have to make sure we're pursuing the right thing. We should look to the present instead of looking to the future. We should focus on doing those tasks that we enjoy and lay the groundwork so that we can do more of it in the future. And we should avoid taking things and people for granted and strive to connect with our friends, loved ones, community and the moment.

If we can do all that, then we should see our personal happiness and our global happiness rise, to from where only a $1/3^{rd}$ of us are very happy, to where unhappiness is the abnormal attribute. We can go from a world where we only talk about the pursuit of happiness to one where happiness becomes a basic human right.

Doesn't that sound lovely? And you can do your part! All you need to do is lead by example. Start off by shifting your focus, changing your habits and finding happiness in your own life. And once your environment sees that it is that easy to make yourself happier, the revolution will spread. How can it not? After all, all of us want to be happy.

And all of us can be.

INSPIRING QUOTES ON HAPPINESS

(A Selection of Some of the Best Quotes About Happiness)

"When one door of happiness closes, another opens, but often we look so long at the closed door that we do not see the one that has been opened for us."
- *Helen Keller -*

⟶✦⟵

"The reason people find it so hard to be happy is that they always see the past better than it was, the present worse than it is, and the future less resolved than it will be."
- *Marcel Pagnol -*

⟶✦⟵

"It isn't what you have, or who you are, or where you are, or what you are doing that makes you happy or unhappy. It is what you think about."
- *Dale Carnegie -*

⟶✦⟵

"True happiness is... to enjoy the present, without anxious dependence upon the future."
- *Lucius Annaeus Seneca -*

"We tend to forget that happiness doesn't come as a result of getting something we don't have, but rather of recognizing and appreciating what we do have."
-   *Frederick Keonig -*

"Success is not the key to happiness. Happiness is the key to success. If you love what you are doing, you will be successful."
-   *Herman Cain -*

"Don't rely on someone else for your happiness and self-worth. Only you can be responsible for that. If you can't love and respect yourself – no one else will be able to make that happen. Accept who you are – completely; the good and the bad – and make changes as YOU see fit – not because you think someone else wants you to be different."
-   *Stacey Charter -*

"Happiness is nothing more than good health and a bad memory."
-    *Albert Schweitzer -*

⊶⊶⊛⊷⊷

Be happy with what you have and are, be generous with both, and you won't have to hunt for happiness.
-    *William E. Gladstone -*

⊶⊶⊛⊷⊷

"Learn to let go. That is the key to happiness."
-    *Buddha -*

⊶⊶⊛⊷⊷

"Happiness is not something ready-made. It comes from your own actions."
-    *Dalai Lama -*

⊶⊶⊛⊷⊷

"If you want happiness for an hour — take a nap.'
 If you want happiness for a day — go fishing.
 If you want happiness for a year — inherit a fortune.
 If you want happiness for a lifetime — help someone else."
-    *Chinese Proverb -*

"Twenty years from now you will be- more disappointed by the things that you didn't do than by the ones you did do. So throw off the bowlines. Sail away from the safe harbor. Catch the trade winds in your sails. Explore. Dream. Discover."
- *Mark Twain -*

"Some cause happiness wherever they go; others whenever they go"
- *Oscar Wilde -*

"Action may not always bring happiness; but there is no happiness without action."
- *Benjamin Disraeli -*

"The secret of happiness is not in doing what one likes, but in liking what one does."
- *James M. Barrie -*

"Of all forms of caution, caution in love is perhaps the most fatal to true happiness."
-   *Bertrand Russell* -

"If you spend your whole life waiting for the storm, you'll never enjoy the sunshine."
-   *Morris West* -

"Everyone wants to live on top of the mountain, but all the happiness and growth occurs while you're climbing it."
-   *Andy Rooney* -

"Being happy doesn't mean everything is perfect. It means you've decided to look beyond the imperfections."
-   *Unknown* -

Infographic: 10 Habits

10 Habits of Happy People

 Habit 1: Acceptance & Perspective

 Habit 2: Giving & Serving

 Habit 3: Relating & Connecting

 Habit 4: Exercise & Health

 Habit 5: Mindfulness & Emotion

 Habit 6: Gratitude & Appreciation

 Habit 7: Do What You Are Good At

 Habit 8: Your Goals & Dreams

 Habit 9: Be Part of Something Bigger

Habit 10: Resilience

Source: 10 Habits of Happy People: Quick & Easy Steps to Be Happy Everyday
(A Practical Guide)
Author: Sofie K

Check Out Other Related Books

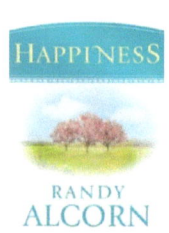

Happiness
Author: Randy Alcorn
ASIN: B00UCEMCXW (Kindle Edition)

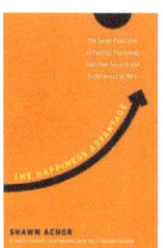

The Happiness Advantage: The Seven
Principles of Positive Psychology That Fuel
Success and Performance at Work
Author: Shawn Achor
ISBN-13: 978-0753539477
ASIN: B003F3PMYI (Kindle Edition)

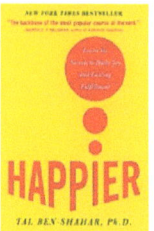

Happier: Learn the Secrets to Daily Joy and
Lasting Fulfillment
Author: Tal Ben-Shahar
ISBN-13: 978-0071543835
ASIN: B003XNTU5M (Kindle Edition)

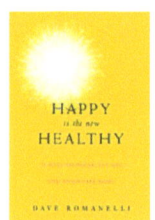

Happy Is the New Healthy: 31 Ways to Relax,
Let Go, and Enjoy Life NOW!
Author: Dave Romanelli
ISBN-13: 978-1629144986
ASIN: B00R3LDW04 (Kindle Edition)

www.ingramcontent.com/pod-product-compliance
Lightning Source LLC
Chambersburg PA
CBHW040325010626
45792CB00024B/2130